HOW TO SLIM DOWN FOR LIFE

A Blueprint to Conquer Obesity

BY DR. LAUREN D. GOLDSTEIN

About The Book

This Book is a guide on building a sustainable and healthy lifestyle. It explores mindset shifts, mindful nutrition, joyful movement, sleep and stress management, supportive relationships, and celebrating progress. It encourages a long-term commitment to well-being, providing practical solutions for each aspect. The goal is to inspire individuals to view health as a continuous journey, fostering habits that endure and contribute to a fulfilling lifestyle.

Disclaimer Notice

Please keep in mind that the information in this book is strictly for educational purposes. Before using any of the codes in this book, please consult a licensed specialist.

Contents

INTRODUCTION

Hey there, fellow traveler on the road to wellness! Buckle up, because you're about to dive into a transformative journey—one that's not just about shedding pounds but reclaiming your health, confidence, and zest for life. Let's kick off this adventure with a hearty welcome and a promise: this won't be your typical weight-loss escapade.

Picture this journey as a thrilling expedition, a blueprint tailor-made for you. It's not about fitting into society's cookie-cutter image; it's about sculpting the best version of yourself. So, lace up those sneakers, grab a water bottle, and let's hit the ground running!

The Reality of Obesity: Facing the Elephant in the Room

Before we delve into the nitty-gritty, let's acknowledge the elephant in the room—obesity. No beating around the bush here. We're diving headfirst into the facts, but fear not, because knowledge is power. Understanding the science behind weight gain and the emotional ties to our eating habits is the compass that'll guide us through uncharted territories.

But hey, we're not here to dwell on the past; we're here to carve out a new narrative—one that empowers, inspires, and leaves behind the weight of yesterday.

Assessing Your Lifestyle: The Starting Point

Now, let's take a pit stop to assess where you're at. Think of it like checking the fuel gauge before a road trip. We'll identify those daily habits, the sneaky triggers that lead to overeating, and together, we'll plot a course for change. Setting realistic goals is the key to success, and we're not aiming for perfection—just progress, one step at a time.

The Blueprint Unveiled: Nutrition, Exercise, and Mindful Living

Our journey's map is divided into sections, and each holds a treasure trove of wisdom. Nutrition becomes your compass, exercise your trusty steed, and mindful living, the wind beneath your wings. We're not just talking diets and workouts; we're talking about crafting a lifestyle that feels as natural as breathing.

Ready to discover the power of a balanced plate, the joy of movement, and the art of savoring each bite? Your blueprint is a personalized guide, not a one-size-fits-all manual.

Navigating Challenges: Plateaus and Social Storms

Ah, but every journey has its challenges, right? Plateaus might feel like detours, but fear not, we'll navigate through and find ways to keep the momentum alive. Social situations? Consider them road bumps, not roadblocks. We'll equip you with strategies to stay on course without missing out on the fun.

The Home Stretch: Building Habits and Celebrating Victories

As we approach the final stretch, it's all about building habits that stand the test of time. This isn't a quick fix; it's a life overhaul. And when you reach that finish line, trust me, the celebration will be epic. Reflect on your journey, embrace the transformation, and bask in the glory of a healthier, happier you.

Your Personalized Blueprint to Lifelong Health: Conclusion

So, my fellow adventurer, this is just the beginning. The journey ahead is exciting, challenging, and entirely yours to conquer. Keep this blueprint close, embrace the changes, and remember, the road to a healthier you is paved with determination, self-love, and a sprinkle of joy.

Are you ready to step into the driver's seat and own this journey? The road awaits, and trust me, the destination is worth every step. Let's roll!

THE REALITY OF OBESITY

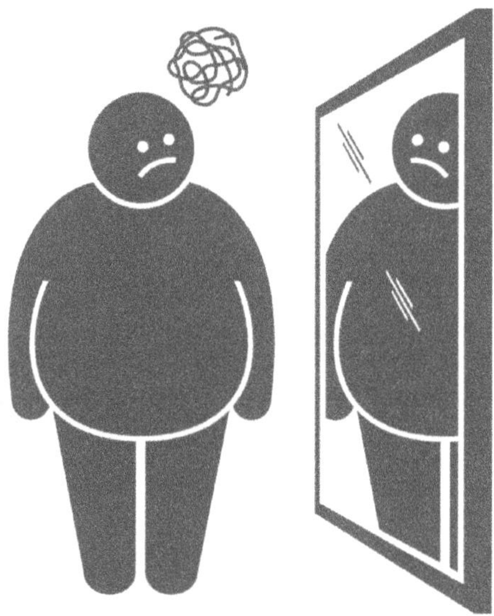

Let's dive deep into a topic that might feel like the elephant in the room, but guess what? We're going to tackle it head-on—no tiptoeing around. Welcome to a conversation about the reality of obesity, a journey that's not about blame but about understanding and taking charge.

Ever wondered why the scale seems to have a mind of its own? Well, it's time to demystify the science behind weight gain. Think of it like uncovering the secret recipe of a dish you've been craving.

Once you know what's cooking, you can start making some changes in your own kitchen.

Now, let's talk emotions. Yep, we're going there. Emotional eating is like having a stormy weather system inside us. But fear not, we've got the umbrella to weather the storm. By unraveling the emotional ties to our eating habits, we're not just addressing the symptoms; we're getting to the root of the issue.

Obesity isn't a character flaw; it's a complex interplay of biology, environment, and emotions. So, let's strip away the judgment, shake off the shame, and face the reality with a newfound understanding.

Sure, we're acknowledging the extra weight in the room, but here's the twist—it's not about dwelling on the past. This journey is about seizing the present, understanding the hows and whys, and crafting a future that's healthier and happier.

So, grab a metaphorical magnifying glass, let's inspect the details, and remember, you're not alone in this exploration. We're in it together, ready to face the reality of obesity with courage, compassion, and a dash of curiosity.

Why Slimming Down Matters

Why slimming down is more than just a numbers game. It's not about chasing an elusive ideal; it's about reclaiming a life that's vibrant, energetic, and uniquely yours.

So, let's kick things off with a simple question: Ever felt like your body was a well-worn suit that just didn't fit quite right? Well, guess what? You're not alone. Slimming down matters because it's about shedding more than just pounds; it's about shedding the discomfort, the fatigue, and the limits that extra weight can place on your life.

Picture this: You're not just losing weight; you're gaining freedom—the freedom to move without hesitation, to embrace activities you love, and to feel a lightness in your step. It's like trading in a heavy backpack for a pair of wings. Slimming down is about unlocking the door to a world of possibilities that might have felt out of reach before.

But it's not just about the physical perks. Slimming down matters because it's a journey that transcends the superficial. It's about boosting confidence, reigniting self-love, and fostering a positive relationship with the incredible vessel that is your body. Imagine your body as a canvas, and each healthy choice you make is a stroke that adds to a masterpiece of well-being.

Now, let's talk energy—because who doesn't want to feel like they've got a turbocharged engine under the hood? Slimming down matters because it's an energy upgrade. It's about reclaiming the vitality that might have taken a back seat amidst the hustle and bustle of life.

And here's the kicker: it's not a one-size-fits-all journey. Your version of slimming down is as unique as your fingerprint. It's about finding what makes you thrive, what fuels your joy, and what aligns with the rhythm of your life.

So, why does slimming down matter? Because it's your ticket to a life that's not just lived but truly embraced. It's about feeling good in your skin, having the energy to savor every moment, and realizing that the journey is just as important as the destination.

Are you ready to embark on this transformative adventure? Your reasons are as valid as your goals, and the beauty lies in the journey itself. Let's make it matter—to you.

SECTION I

UNDERSTANDING OBESITY

CHAPTER I

BREAKING DOWN OBESITY

Health explorer! we're on a mission to demystify the heavyweight champion in the room—obesity. It's not just about numbers on a scale; it's about understanding the science, the why behind the what. So, buckle up for a journey into the intricacies of breaking down obesity.

Let's start with a question: Ever felt like your body was speaking a language you couldn't quite decipher? That's the science of weight gain, my friend. It's like peeling back the layers of a complex novel to reveal the plot twists. We're decoding the signals, understanding how our bodies store and use energy, and unraveling the mystery of why shedding those extra pounds isn't always as simple as "eat less, move more."

Think of it like a chemistry experiment. We're mixing variables—genetics, environment, and lifestyle—and observing the reactions. It's not a one-size-fits-all equation; it's a unique cocktail for each of us. Understanding this personalized formula is the key to unlocking the door to a healthier you.

Now, let's talk metabolism—the superhero in our body's saga. Sometimes it works in mysterious ways, slowing down or speeding up based on various factors. It's not about blaming metabolism; it's about befriending it, understanding its quirks, and figuring out how to make it your ally in the battle against extra pounds.

But here's the twist: breaking down obesity isn't just a solo mission. It's a dynamic duo of biology and behavior. We're not just addressing the physical aspects; we're diving into the emotional ties to food, the stressors that can tip the scales, and the habits that become the building blocks of our health.

Picture it like a puzzle—each piece representing a facet of your journey. We're putting together the puzzle of your body, understanding how the pieces fit, and creating a clear picture of a healthier, happier you.

So, why break down obesity? Because it's not just about shedding weight; it's about gaining knowledge, empowerment, and control. It's about rewriting the narrative, moving from frustration to understanding, and embracing the fact that your body is a unique masterpiece.

Ready to be the detective in your own health story? Let's break it down together, piece by piece, until we uncover the path to a healthier, happier you. The adventure begins now!

THE SCIENCE BEHIND WEIGHT GAIN

The intricate dance our bodies perform that goes beyond just the numbers on the scale. Think of it as unraveling the plot twists of a captivating novel, where every chapter is a piece of the puzzle called **"The Science Behind Weight Gain."**

So, let's start with the basics. Ever felt like your body was speaking a language you couldn't quite understand? That's the body's way of communicating the science of weight gain. It's like deciphering the secret code to our own unique story. We're talking about the incredible orchestra of hormones, genetics, and lifestyle choices that influence the scale's numbers.

Now, picture this: your body as a high-tech chemistry lab. We're mixing elements like genetics and environment, observing the reactions, and understanding how they contribute to the weight gain equation. It's not a cookie-cutter formula; it's a personalized concoction for each of us.

Metabolism, the superhero of our body's saga, plays a leading role. It's not just about blaming a sluggish metabolism; it's about understanding its quirks and turning it into your sidekick in the battle against weight gain. Metabolism is like the conductor of this symphony, dictating the tempo of our energy expenditure.

But here's the twist—it's not just about the biological ballet. The emotional ties to food, the stressors that tip the scales, and the daily habits that become the rhythm of our lives are also part of the narrative. It's a dynamic duo of biology and behavior, and understanding both is key to creating a harmony that leads to a healthier weight.

Imagine weight gain as a puzzle. Each piece represents a facet of your journey. We're not just putting together the puzzle of your body; we're creating a clear picture of how to navigate the path to a healthier, more balanced you.

So, why delve into the science behind weight gain? Because it's not just about shedding pounds; it's about gaining knowledge, empowerment, and control. It's about rewriting the narrative, moving from confusion to understanding, and embracing the fact that your body is a unique masterpiece.

Ready to embark on this scientific adventure? Let's unravel the complexities, decode the mysteries, and rewrite the story of your body's journey. The science of weight gain awaits, and you're the protagonist in this epic tale!

THE MYTH OF "PERFECT" BODY WEIGHT

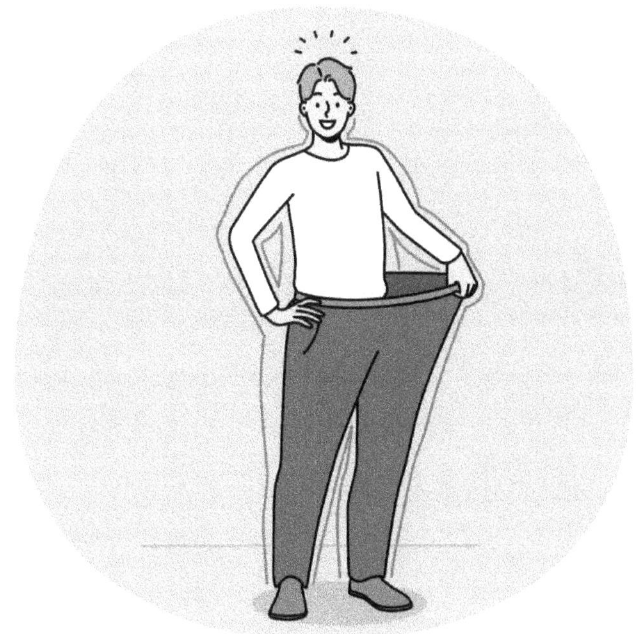

Spoiler alert: there's no one-size-fits-all when it comes to the ideal weight, and we're here to unravel the myth, redefine the narrative, and liberate you from the shackles of unrealistic standards.

First things first, have you ever wondered who decides what the "perfect" body weight is? It's like chasing a mirage in the desert—always there but never quite within reach. The truth is, there's no universal definition of perfection when it comes to our bodies. It's like trying to fit everyone into the same pair of jeans—uncomfortable and downright impossible.

Let's break it down. The myth of the "perfect" body weight often stems from external influences, societal pressures, and a barrage of images that scream, "This is the ideal." But here's the reality check: your body is not a mannequin meant to conform to someone else's idea of beauty or health. It's a dynamic, unique entity that deserves to be celebrated for its individuality.

Now, let's talk health. Picture this: a garden with diverse flowers of all shapes and sizes. Just like no two flowers are identical, no two bodies are the same. Health is not a one-size-fits-all equation. It's about nourishing your body, feeling energetic, and enjoying a life that's fulfilling. It's not about squeezing into a predetermined mold but finding the shape that allows you to bloom.

The myth of the "perfect" body weight can lead to a never-ending cycle of frustration, comparison, and self-doubt. It's like chasing a rainbow without realizing that the pot of gold is right where you are. Instead of fixating on a number on the scale, let's shift the focus to how you feel—energetic, confident, and comfortable in your skin.

So, why unravel this myth? Because it's time to embrace the beauty of diversity, to celebrate the uniqueness of your body, and to redefine health on your terms. It's about breaking free from the chains of societal expectations and stepping into a realm where happiness and well-being take center stage.

Are you ready to let go of the myth and embrace the reality of your amazing, one-of-a-kind self? The journey to health and happiness begins when you toss aside the illusion of perfection and start appreciating the masterpiece that is you. Let's redefine the narrative and make your story one of self-love and authenticity.

CHAPTER 2

EMOTIONAL CONNECTION TO WEIGHT

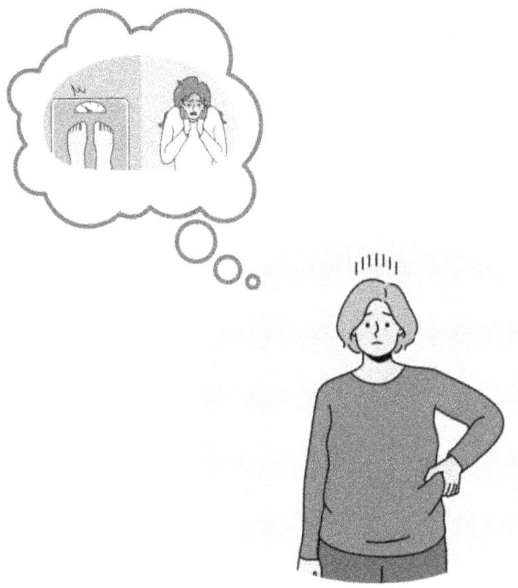

A journey where our feelings and food become dance partners, twirling through the highs and lows of our lives. It's like weaving a tapestry of emotions, and sometimes, the threads get a bit tangled.

Ever caught yourself reaching for that chocolate bar when stress comes knocking? Or finding solace in a bowl of ice cream after a tough day? That's the emotional connection to weight at play. It's not just about satisfying hunger; it's about using food as a companion, a confidante, or a comforting hug.

Let's picture it like a relationship status on social media: "It's complicated." Our emotions and our eating habits are entwined, each influencing the other. It's not a simple equation of calories in and calories out; it's a dynamic dance between our mood and our meals.

Now, let's talk comfort food. Have you ever had a rough day and found refuge in a dish that reminds you of home? It's like wrapping yourself in a warm blanket of memories. But here's the twist—comfort food doesn't always have to be synonymous with unhealthy choices. It's about finding alternatives that nurture your soul without compromising your health.

On the flip side, stress eating is like a storm that sweeps through, leaving behind a trail of wrappers and regret. The solution? It's not about banishing stress from your life—that's as impossible as controlling the weather. It's about finding healthier coping mechanisms, like a sturdy umbrella that shields you from the downpour of emotional eating.

And then there's the joyous celebration indulgence. Ever found yourself feasting in moments of happiness? It's like raising a toast with your taste buds. But the key is balance—celebration doesn't have to translate to a food free-for-all. It's about savoring the joy without drowning it in excess.

Now, let's talk solutions. Instead of viewing emotions and food as frenemies, what if we transformed them into allies? Picture it like a tag team—your emotions guiding you to make mindful food choices, and food becoming a source of nourishment for both body and soul.

Mindful eating is like a compass in this emotional landscape. It's about savoring each bite, listening to your body's cues, and being present in the moment. When you tune into your emotions without judgment, you're equipped to make choices that honor both your feelings and your well-being.

So, why explore the emotional connection to weight? Because understanding this intricate relationship is the key to a balanced and healthier lifestyle. It's about untangling the threads, redefining the way we view food, and creating a space where emotions and eating coexist harmoniously.

EXPLORING EMOTIONAL EATING

An intricate dance between our feelings and the fridge. It's like sailing through the seas of emotion, and sometimes, we find ourselves in stormy waters where food becomes our anchor.

Have you ever reached for a tub of ice cream after a tough day, thinking it would be the cure-all for stress? Or maybe indulged in a bag of chips during a Netflix binge, only to realize you've eaten the entire thing without even noticing? That, my friend, is the realm of emotional eating. It's not about hunger; it's about using food to cope with our emotions, whether it's joy, sadness, stress, or boredom.

Imagine your emotions as a roller coaster, and food as the tempting cotton candy stand at the amusement park. Emotional eating is like hopping on that roller coaster without realizing you're in for a loop-de-loop of guilt and regret afterward. It's a common coping mechanism, but the tricky part is finding healthier ways to navigate the twists and turns of our feelings.

Now, let's talk solutions. Picture this: you're stressed out, and the vending machine is calling your name. Instead of reaching for that candy bar, take a detour to the park for a brisk walk. Exercise is like a superhero cape, ready to rescue you from the clutches of emotional eating. It releases feel-good endorphins that can lift your mood without the side effects of a sugar crash.

Another scenario: boredom strikes, and the pantry seems like the only exciting place. How about swapping that bag of chips for a creative activity? Engaging your mind in a hobby or a project can be a powerful distraction from the munchies. It's like finding treasure in the backyard instead of raiding the snack drawer.

The key is to tune into your emotions and ask yourself, "Am I truly hungry, or is there something else going on?" It's like becoming the detective of your own feelings, unraveling the mystery of why you're reaching for that comfort food. Journaling can be a fantastic tool—scribble down your emotions, and you might discover patterns that lead to healthier choices.

So, why explore emotional eating? Because understanding the connection between feelings and food is the first step toward building a healthier relationship with both. It's about transforming the roller coaster ride into a gentle sail, where you navigate the seas of emotion with mindfulness and self-compassion.

OVERCOMING PSYCHOLOGICAL BARRIERS

We're stepping into the battlefield of the mind, addressing those pesky psychological barriers that can feel like heavy chains holding us back. It's like entering a maze where our thoughts play the role of both the walls and the escape route. But fear not, because we're about to navigate through and emerge victorious on the other side.

Ever felt like your mind was playing tricks on you, convincing you that certain goals are out of reach? It's like having a skilled illusionist performing in the theater of your thoughts. These psychological barriers can be as subtle as whispers or as loud as a roaring crowd, telling you that you're not capable, not worthy, or that success is an impossible dream.

Now, let's tackle the first barrier: self-doubt. Have you ever hesitated to take that first step because a little voice inside said, "What if you fail?" It's like standing at the edge of a diving board, contemplating the plunge. But here's the truth bomb—failure is not the end; it's a stepping stone. Embrace it, learn from it, and use it as fuel for your journey.

Next up, fear of the unknown. It's like staring into a pitch-black cave, uncertain of what lies ahead. But guess what? The unknown is where magic happens. Instead of fearing it, let curiosity be your lantern, guiding you through the shadows. Every step into the unknown is a step closer to growth and discovery.

And let's not forget the comparison trap. Ever scrolled through social media and felt like everyone else has it figured out except you? It's like being in a race without a finish line. But here's the reality check—everyone's journey is unique. Focus on your path, your progress, and celebrate the small victories. Comparison is the thief of joy; don't let it rob you of your successes.

Now, let's talk solutions. Imagine your psychological barriers as a wall of fog. Instead of waiting for it to lift, take a step forward. Action is your fog light, gradually revealing the path. Break down your goals into manageable steps, creating a staircase that leads you over the barriers.

And here's a secret weapon: positive affirmations. It's like giving your mind a pep talk. Replace the negative whispers with affirmations that boost your confidence and shift your mindset. The mind is a powerful ally when you choose to be its captain.

So, why overcome these psychological barriers? Because the life you want is on the other side, and the only thing standing between you and it is the maze of your thoughts. It's about reclaiming control, rewriting the script, and realizing that you are the author of your story.

SECTION 2

SETTING THE FOUNDATION

CHAPTER 3

ASSESSING YOUR CURRENT LIFESTYLE

A journey of self-discovery, a bit like taking out a magnifying glass and examining the daily habits that shape our lives. Welcome to the crucial checkpoint in your well-being adventure—assessing your current lifestyle.

First off, have you ever felt like your days are on autopilot, rushing through the motions without a moment to catch your breath? It's like being on a train with no clear destination. Assessing your current lifestyle is like pulling the emergency brake and taking a moment to look around, to understand where you are and where you want to go.

Now, let's talk daily habits. Think of them as the building blocks of your life—the choices you make every day that shape your well-being. It's not about perfection; it's about progress. Whether it's the snack you grab during a mid-afternoon slump or the way you unwind before bedtime, these habits paint a picture of your current lifestyle.

Consider this: assessing your lifestyle is like taking an inventory of your toolkit before a big adventure. What habits are serving you well, and which ones might need a little recalibration? Maybe it's that extra cup of sugary coffee in the morning or the habit of scrolling through social media before bed. Identifying these habits is the first step to creating positive change.

Now, let's talk solutions. It's not about making drastic overhauls overnight; that's like trying to sprint a marathon. Instead, consider small tweaks that align with your well-being goals. Maybe swap that sugary coffee for a revitalizing herbal tea in the morning or replace late-night screen time with a chapter of a good book.

Setting realistic and achievable goals is like charting the course for your well-being adventure. It's not about aiming for an unattainable summit but about choosing paths that lead to long-term success. Celebrate the small wins along the way—they're like trail markers guiding you toward a healthier, happier you.

And here's a powerful tool: mindfulness. It's like having a compass in your pocket. Pay attention to how your habits make you feel. Are they energizing or draining? Mindfulness helps you navigate the terrain of your lifestyle with awareness and intention.

So, why assess your current lifestyle? Because understanding where you are is the compass that guides you to where you want to be. It's about taking the reins, steering your well-being adventure with purpose, and crafting a life that aligns with your values and goals.

Ready to take that magnifying glass to your daily habits? The adventure awaits, and you're the protagonist. Assess, tweak, celebrate, and watch as your well-being journey unfolds. Let's set sail into a lifestyle that feels not just lived but truly embraced. The compass is in your hands—let the adventure begin!

DAILY HABITS IMPACTING YOUR WEIGHT

Imagine your body is like a garden, and every day, you have little habits that are like the seeds you plant in that garden. These habits, just like the seeds, can affect how your garden grows, and in this case, it's about how your body feels and looks.

So, let's talk about these daily habits impacting your weight. Think of them as the way you water and take care of your garden every single day. Some habits can be like giving your garden the right amount of sunshine and nutrients, making it grow healthy and strong. These are habits that can help you maintain a weight that feels good for you.

Now, picture this: if you water your garden with soda instead of water, or if you only give it candy instead of fruits and veggies, what do you think will happen? Your garden might not grow as well, right? That's how certain habits, like drinking sugary drinks or eating too many sweets, can impact your body and maybe make it a bit heavier than you'd like.

On the flip side, if you make a habit of playing outside and eating yummy fruits and veggies, it's like giving your garden the best care possible. Those habits can help your body feel energized and happy, just like a garden that's full of colorful and vibrant flowers.

Let's talk about moving around—imagine playing tag, riding your bike, or dancing. These are habits that can make your body strong and active, just like how running and playing can make your garden lively and full of life.

So, in a nutshell, daily habits impacting your weight are the little things you do every day that either help your garden (body) grow beautifully or maybe make it a bit tricky for the flowers to bloom. Choosing habits like eating healthy foods and being active is like being a superhero for your garden, ensuring it thrives and stays amazing!

IDENTIFYING TRIGGERS FOR OVEREATING

Have you ever thought of a situation where your tummy is like a treasure chest, and you want to make sure it stays happy and doesn't get too full of snacks. Identifying triggers for overeating is like being a detective and figuring out what makes you want to eat more than your tummy really needs.

So, let's talk about triggers. Triggers are like little clues or signals that make you think, "Hmm, I want to eat something!" They can be sneaky, like when you feel sad, bored, or even when you see your favorite cartoon on TV.

Picture this: if every time you feel a bit sad, you want to eat cookies, that's a trigger! The sadness is like a flag waving, telling you, "Time for cookies!" But here's the secret detective part – you can find other ways to comfort yourself when you're sad, like hugging your teddy bear or drawing a happy picture.

Another trigger can be when you see a big bowl of colorful candies. Your eyes get all sparkly, and suddenly, you really, really want to eat them. That's a trigger too! But you can be a super smart detective and choose to have just a few candies or maybe save them for a special treat.

So, identifying triggers for overeating is like having a special map that helps you understand why you feel like eating. Once you know your triggers, you can make choices that keep your tummy happy and your treasure chest of snacks just right. It's like being the captain of your own food adventure, making sure your tummy and your body feel amazing!

CHAPTER 4

GOAL SETTING FOR SUCCESS

Illustration

Let's imagine you're the captain of your very own spaceship, and you want to fly it to the moon because that's your big, exciting goal! Goal setting for success is like making a super-duper plan to reach the moon and have an awesome adventure.

First, you need to decide exactly where on the moon you want to go. Do you want to land in a crater, bounce around on the surface, or maybe even discover space rocks? That's setting a specific goal, like deciding the exact spot you want to explore.

Now, you need to figure out how to get there. Do you need a super-fast rocket or a magical spaceship with wings? That's setting a measurable goal, like knowing how fast or how far you need to go to reach your moon destination.

But wait, it's not just about the spaceship. You also need to pack the right snacks and wear a cool space suit, right? That's setting achievable goals, like making sure you have all the tools and skills you need for your moon mission.

And here's the cool part – you can't just stare at the moon and hope to get there. You need to start the engines, count down, and blast off! That's setting realistic goals, like taking small steps that actually get you closer to your big goal.

But what if you get a little lost in space or encounter space monsters? That's where having a friend, like Mission Control, comes in handy. Setting time-bound goals means giving yourself a deadline, like saying, "I'll reach the moon in two weeks." This way, you stay focused and have a space buddy to help you along the way.

So, goal setting for success is like being the hero of your own space adventure, deciding where you want to go, planning how to get there, making sure you have everything you need, and counting down to launch! Whether it's exploring the moon or achieving other big dreams, setting goals is like having your very own treasure map to success!

ESTABLISHING REALISTIC AND ACHIEVABLE GOALS

Achievable goals is like plotting the course for your own epic journey. Whether you're aiming for the moon or just trying to conquer the everyday mountains, establishing realistic and achievable goals is your trusty compass. So, grab your imaginary map, and let's dive into the world of goal-setting!

Imagine you're the captain of a ship, sailing across the vast sea of possibilities. Your destination? A magical island called Success. Now, before you set sail, it's crucial to decide exactly where on the island you want to go. Do you fancy a stroll through the Enchanted Forest or a dip in the Sea of Accomplishments? Setting a specific goal is like marking that "X" on your treasure map, giving your journey a clear direction.

But hold on, Captain! Knowing where to go is just the first step. Picture your ship with its sails billowing in the wind—that's your goal taking shape. Now, let's make it measurable. How fast do you want to sail, and how many days until you reach the shores of Success? Making your goal measurable is like setting the coordinates on your ship's navigation system, ensuring you stay on course.

Now, it's time to pack your bags for the voyage. Think of achievable goals as choosing the right tools for your journey. Do you need a sturdy anchor for challenges, a compass for guidance, or a telescope to spot opportunities on the horizon? Making sure your bags are filled with achievable tools sets you up for a smooth sailing experience.

But, my fellow adventurer, remember that even the bravest captains encounter storms. That's where setting realistic goals comes into play. It's like adjusting your sails to navigate through rough waters, acknowledging that the journey might have twists and turns, but you're equipped to handle them.

Now, let's talk deadlines—a bit like giving yourself a treasure map with a big "X" marking the date of your arrival on Success Island. Having a time-bound goal adds urgency and excitement to your journey. It's not about rushing but ensuring that you're steadily making progress toward your destination.

So, why embark on the quest of setting realistic and achievable goals? Because it transforms your journey into a purposeful adventure. It's about being the hero of your story, navigating through uncharted waters, and celebrating victories along the way. Your ship, your map, your adventure—setting goals is the wind in your sails, propelling you toward a horizon filled with triumphs and treasures.

Ready to hoist the anchor and set sail? Your adventure awaits, and each goal you set is a step closer to the island of Success. So, fellow explorer, grab your map, unfurl your sails, and let's chart a course toward a future filled with achievements and discoveries! The sea of possibilities is calling, and you're the master of your own destiny. Bon voyage!

SECTION 3

THE BLUEPRINT TO SLIMMING DOWN

CHAPTER 5

NUTRITION ESSENTIALS

Think of it as a grand feast for your body, a menu filled with nutrients that fuel your energy and keep you shining like a star. So, grab your fork and knife, and let's delve into the delightful world of nourishment!

Picture your body as a high-tech spaceship, zooming through the vastness of space. Every part of this spaceship requires special fuel to function at its best, and that fuel comes from the food we eat. Now, think about nutrients as the cosmic energy that powers your ship. They come in different forms, each playing a crucial role in keeping your body systems running smoothly.

First up, we have protein—the building blocks of your spaceship. It's like the sturdy foundation that holds everything together. Whether it's repairing damaged parts or building new ones, protein is the superhero that ensures your spaceship stays strong and resilient.

Next on the menu is carbohydrates—the rocket fuel of your culinary spacecraft. They provide the energy needed for takeoff, ensuring your daily activities are smooth and steady. Just like a rocket needs fuel to reach new heights, your body relies on carbohydrates to power through the day.

Now, let's talk about fats—the cosmic cushion for your spaceship. Imagine fats as the cozy blankets that keep your systems snug and warm. They provide insulation, support organ function, and even act as messengers for important signals within your body. It's about choosing the right kind of fats to ensure your spaceship stays well-insulated without getting weighed down.

Don't forget about vitamins and minerals—the celestial navigators of your culinary journey. They're like the star maps that guide your spaceship through the vast galaxy of well-being. From vitamin C, the guardian of your immune system, to calcium, the protector of your bone health, these micronutrients play vital roles in keeping your ship on the right course.

And of course, there's water—the cosmic elixir that keeps your spaceship hydrated and ready for any adventure. It's like the fueling station on a distant planet, ensuring you stay refreshed and energized throughout your culinary expedition.

So, why delve into the realm of nutrition essentials? Because understanding the cosmic menu of nutrients empowers you to make choices that elevate your well-being. It's about crafting a culinary journey that not only satisfies your taste buds but also nourishes your body, making your spaceship the envy of the galaxy.

Ready to embark on this culinary odyssey? Grab your cosmic cookbook, choose nutrient-rich ingredients, and let's create a menu that propels you toward a future filled with energy, vitality, and the joy of culinary exploration. May your plates be bountiful, and your journey through the galaxy of nutrition be as thrilling as a warp-speed adventure!

Weekly Checkout

Activities	Week 1	Week 2	Week 3	Week 4	Week 5	Week 6	Week 7
Initial Weight							
Weight Loss							

BUILDING A BALANCED PLATE

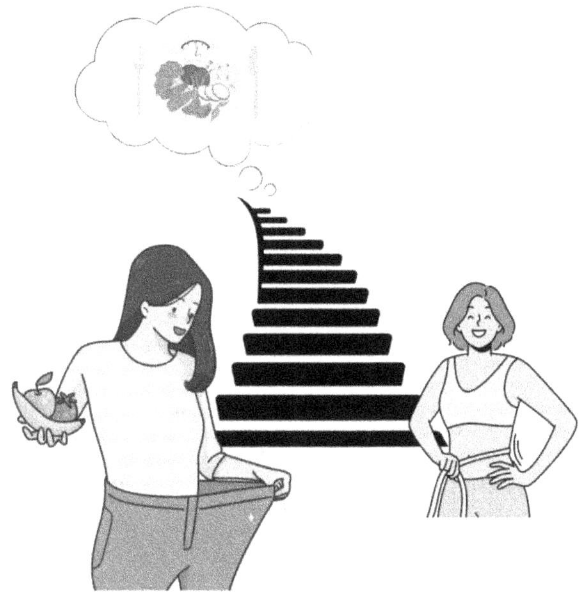

Imagine your plate as a canvas, and the ingredients as your vibrant palette of colors, each contributing to a masterpiece that not only tantalizes your taste buds but also nourishes your body. Let's embark on this culinary journey together and explore the secrets of crafting a balanced and delectable plate.

First things first, let's talk about the stars of your culinary show—proteins, the bold brushstrokes that form the foundation of your plate. Whether it's the lean elegance of grilled chicken or the robust richness of legumes, proteins are the protagonists that add substance and depth to your gastronomic canvas. They are the builders, laying the groundwork for a satiating and satisfying culinary experience.

Next up, we have carbohydrates—the lively hues that infuse energy and vitality into your plate. Picture them as the sunshine-yellow accents that brighten up your canvas. Whether it's the wholesome grains, the playful potatoes, or the vibrant veggies, carbohydrates bring a burst of life, providing the fuel your body needs for its daily adventures.

Now, let's add a touch of greenery—vegetables, the verdant strokes that bring freshness and vibrancy to your culinary masterpiece. They're like the lush foliage in a garden, offering an array of textures and flavors. From crisp greens to colorful bell peppers, vegetables not only enhance the visual appeal but also contribute essential nutrients, making your plate a celebration of health and flavor.

Enter fats—the subtle shadows that add depth and richness to your composition. Like a skilled artist using shading techniques, you can choose healthy fats, such as avocado or olive oil, to impart a silky smoothness to your plate. Fats not only enhance the overall taste but also play a crucial role in supporting various bodily functions.

And let's not forget the seasoning—herbs and spices, the magical elements that elevate your culinary creation to a symphony of flavors. Think of them as the notes in a melody, adding a harmonious blend of tastes and aromas. Whether it's the warmth of cinnamon, the zing of cilantro, or the savory embrace of garlic, these culinary accents transform your plate into a sensory delight.

Now, the question arises—why strive for a balanced plate? Well, it's about creating a culinary masterpiece that not only delights your taste buds but also provides your body with the essential nutrients it craves. It's the art of nourishing yourself, a daily ritual that contributes to your overall well-being.

So, let's pick up our culinary brushes and embark on the adventure of building a balanced plate. Consider your plate a canvas, and each ingredient a stroke of creativity. Play with colors, textures, and flavors, allowing your culinary instincts to guide you. Craft a plate that not only satisfies your cravings but also leaves you feeling nourished and invigorated—a true masterpiece on your gastronomic canvas. Happy creating!

NAVIGATING DIETS: WHAT WORKS AND WHAT DOESN'T

First mate on this voyage is the "One-Size-Fits-All" diet. It's like a pre-made compass that claims to work for everyone. But here's the catch—our bodies are unique, like individual ships with their own needs and preferences. What sails smoothly for one might hit rough waters for another. It's crucial to recognize that a diet tailored to your specific needs and lifestyle is your trusty North Star.

Now, let's set our sights on the "Quick-Fix Island" diet. It promises speedy treasures in the form of rapid weight loss. But beware, this island might be filled with hidden dangers. Quick fixes often lack the sustainability needed for long-term well-being. It's like setting sail without enough supplies—eventually, the ship might run aground. Opting for gradual changes and sustainable habits is like charting a course with a steady breeze, ensuring a smoother and more lasting journey.

Ah, the "No-Fun Allowed" diet, a treacherous territory where joy in eating becomes a distant memory. It's like sailing through murky waters without the sun on your face. Food is not just fuel; it's an integral part of our human experience. A successful diet embraces both health and happiness. Picture it as a ship adorned with colorful flags, sailing under the banner of both nutrition and enjoyment.

Let's not forget the "Extreme Restriction" diet, where certain food groups are banished like pirates from the ship. It might seem like a bold strategy, but cutting out essential nutrients is like poking holes in the hull. Balance is key. A diverse diet ensures you receive a full spectrum of nutrients, keeping your ship sturdy and resilient.

On the brighter side, the "Mindful Eating" approach is like a gentle breeze guiding your ship. It encourages savoring each bite, listening to your body's cues, and enjoying a variety of foods. It's about building a healthy relationship with food, creating a voyage where satisfaction and nourishment coexist harmoniously.

So, why navigate diets at all? Because finding the right course impacts not only your physical well-being but also your mental and emotional health. It's about discovering a diet that aligns with your lifestyle, preferences, and health goals—a voyage that leads to a balanced and fulfilling life.

As you chart your course through the sea of diets, remember to be the captain of your ship. Tailor your approach, seek balance, and enjoy the journey. The culinary seas are vast, and with a well-navigated diet, you're equipped to sail toward a horizon of health, happiness, and culinary delight. Bon voyage!

CHAPTER 6

THE POWER OF PHYSICAL ACTIVITY

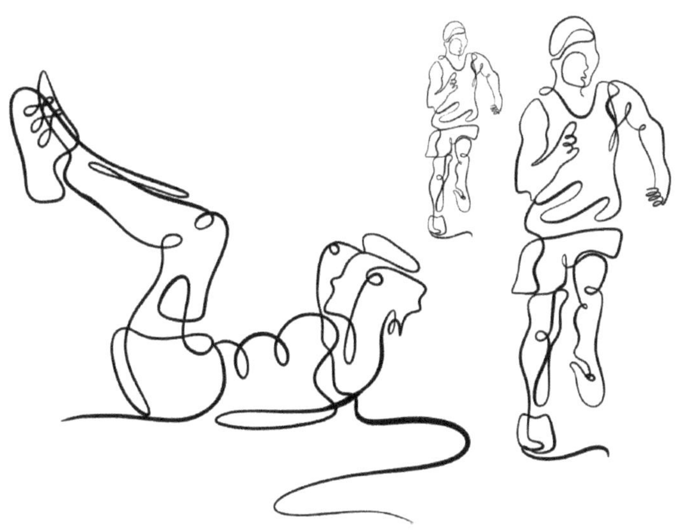

Picture your body as a fortress, and physical activity as the guardian knight, standing tall and ready for action. It's not just about breaking a sweat; it's about empowering your fortress with the strength to face challenges head-on. So, why is physical activity the true superhero in our story?

First and foremost, let's talk about the heart, our body's courageous leader. Physical activity is like a grand ball for the heart, where it dances and strengthens its mighty muscles. With each beat, it's not just maintaining rhythm; it's practicing a powerful battle cry against the foes of cardiovascular issues. It's the heartbeat of a hero, pumping vitality through the entire kingdom of your body.

But the wonders of physical activity don't stop there. Imagine your lungs as the sturdy bellows of a blacksmith's forge. When you engage in physical activity, it's like giving those bellows a good workout, expanding their capacity and enhancing the efficiency of the oxygen exchange. It's the breath of a warrior, fueling your body with the life force it craves.

Now, let's talk about the powerhouse of your fortress—the muscles. Physical activity is the master architect, sculpting and strengthening these powerhouses. It's not just about aesthetics; it's about creating a resilient fortress that can withstand the tests of time. It's the muscles flexing their might, ready to tackle the challenges that come your way.

But here's the magical twist—physical activity is not just about the body; it's a potion that elevates the mind. It's like a wizard's spell, releasing endorphins, the enchanting neurotransmitters that bring forth feelings of joy and reduce stress. It's the magic wand that clears the fog from your mental landscape, leaving you with clarity and a sense of accomplishment.

Now, imagine your body as a treasure chest, and physical activity as the golden key. It unlocks a treasure trove of benefits—improved mood, enhanced sleep, and a bolstered immune system. It's not just a routine; it's the journey to uncover the riches of well-being and vitality.

So, how can you tap into this superhero power? It's not about donning a cape; it's about finding activities that bring you joy. Whether it's dancing like nobody's watching, embracing the serenity of yoga, or venturing into the great outdoors for a refreshing walk, the key is to make it an adventure, not a chore.

In conclusion, the power of physical activity is a force to be reckoned with—a true superhero in our daily narrative. It's not about adhering to strict regimens; it's about embracing movement as a celebration of life. So, fellow adventurers, lace up those metaphorical boots, wield the sword of joyous activities, and let the superhero within you emerge. The journey to a healthier, happier, and more vibrant life begins with a single step. Onward!

FINDING AN EXERCISE ROUTINE YOU LOVE

The enchanted forest where we seek not just physical strength, but the joy that comes from moving our bodies in ways that make our hearts sing. It's time to find an exercise routine that's not a chore but a delightful journey.

Think of your body as a grand playground, and exercise as the magical games you get to play. The key to a successful exercise routine is not about lifting weights with a scowl or running on a treadmill with a heavy heart. It's about finding the game that lights a spark in your eyes, the dance that makes your soul groove, or the adventure that turns your workout into a quest.

Let's debunk the myth that exercise has to be a grueling task. Imagine it's like choosing your favorite flavor of ice cream. There are countless options, and the goal is to find the one that makes you go, "Yes, this is it!" Whether it's the joy of swimming, the zen of yoga, or the thrill of a dance class, the treasure chest of fitness awaits, and you get to pick the golden key.

Have you ever noticed that when you're doing something you love, time seems to fly by? That's the magic of finding an exercise routine that resonates with your soul. It's not about counting down the minutes until it's over; it's about savoring every moment, like a delightful chapter in your favorite book or a scene from a movie that you never want to end.

Now, let's talk about the benefits beyond the physical. Exercise is not just a sculptor of muscles; it's a painter of moods and emotions.

It's the artist that transforms stress into a masterpiece of serenity, anxiety into a canvas of calmness, and fatigue into a portrait of renewed energy. Finding an exercise routine you love is like discovering a secret garden where both your body and mind can bloom.

But how do you unearth this treasure? It's about experimenting, trying out different activities, and paying attention to what makes your heart race with excitement. Do you enjoy the feeling of wind in your hair as you cycle through the neighborhood? Or does the rhythm of music make your feet itch to dance? The key is to let curiosity guide you, like a compass pointing toward the undiscovered lands of joyful movement.

In conclusion, finding an exercise routine you love is not just a journey; it's a grand adventure. It's about turning your workout into a celebration of what your body can do and reveling in the joy of movement. So, fellow explorers, lace up your sneakers, grab your metaphorical map, and set forth into the enchanted forest of fitness. The treasure of a healthier, happier you awaits, and the path to it is filled with the magic of exercises you truly adore. Happy exploring!

Incorporating a variety of exercises into your routine can be a great way to combat obesity. Remember to consult with a healthcare professional or fitness expert before starting any new exercise program, especially if you have existing health concerns. Here's a list of exercises that can help in reducing obesity and a brief on how to perform them:

1. **Walking:**

   - **How to:** Start with a brisk walk for at least 30 minutes a day. You can gradually increase your pace and duration as your fitness improves.

2. **Running or Jogging:**

- **How to:** Begin with a light jog and gradually increase your speed. You can choose outdoor trails or use a treadmill for convenience.

3. **Cycling:**

   - **How to:** Whether it's a stationary bike or cycling outdoors, aim for at least 30 minutes of moderate cycling. Adjust the resistance to challenge yourself.

4. **Swimming:**

   - **How to:** Swim laps in a pool or take water aerobics classes. Swimming is a low-impact exercise that engages multiple muscle groups.

5. **Strength Training:**

   - **How to:** Incorporate weightlifting or bodyweight exercises like squats, lunges, and push-ups. Start with lighter weights and gradually increase as your strength improves.

6. **High-Intensity Interval Training (HIIT):**

   - **How to:** Alternate between short bursts of intense exercise (like sprinting or jumping jacks) and periods of rest. This boosts metabolism and burns calories effectively.

7. **Yoga:**

   - **How to:** Practice yoga poses that engage different muscle groups. It not only helps in physical fitness but also promotes mental well-being.

8. **Pilates:**

- **How to:** Focus on core strength and stability through controlled movements. Pilates is excellent for building overall body strength.

9. **Dance Workouts:**

   - **How to:** Join dance classes or follow online dance workouts. Dancing is a fun way to burn calories and improve cardiovascular health.

10. **Elliptical Training:**

    - **How to:** Use an elliptical machine for a low-impact, full-body workout. Adjust the resistance to challenge yourself.

11. **Rowing:**

    - **How to:** Whether on a rowing machine or out on a boat, rowing engages both upper and lower body muscles.

12. **Aerobic Exercises:**

    - **How to:** Include aerobic exercises like jumping jacks, skipping rope, or aerobics classes to elevate your heart rate.

Remember, consistency is key. Start gradually, listen to your body, and progressively increase the intensity. It's also important to combine exercise with a balanced diet for optimal results in your journey towards a healthier lifestyle.

CHAPTER 7

MINDFUL EATING

One that goes beyond simply eating and dives into the art of mindful indulgence. Think of it as unwrapping a gift, slowly and with intention, revealing the true essence of flavors, textures, and the joy that every bite brings.

In our fast-paced world, where meals are often wolfed down like a sprint, the concept of mindful eating acts as a gentle reminder to hit the brakes. It's not about counting calories or following rigid diets; it's about transforming the act of eating into a sensory experience, a symphony where every bite plays a note.

Consider your plate as a canvas, and each dish as a unique masterpiece waiting to be explored. Mindful eating encourages us to engage all our senses in this culinary adventure. How does the food look? What aromas are dancing in the air? How does it feel against the tongue? It's about being fully present, creating a connection between you and your plate that goes beyond mere consumption.

Picture yourself in a serene garden, surrounded by the vibrant colors and scents of nature. Mindful eating is akin to savoring a delicious fruit picked straight from the tree—the crisp snap of an apple, the juicy burst of a grape. It's about relishing each sensation, cultivating a mindful relationship with what you consume.

Ever find yourself munching absentmindedly in front of the TV or while scrolling through your phone? Mindful eating gently nudges us to break free from these autopilot eating habits. It's about turning off the distractions, tuning into your body's hunger cues, and appreciating the act of nourishing yourself without the noise of external stimuli.

Let's not forget the magic of chewing. Yes, something as simple as chewing. It's not just a mechanical process; it's the first step in the digestive ballet. Mindful eating encourages us to chew slowly, allowing the flavors to unfold, and sending signals to the brain that, "Hey, we're eating!" This conscious chewing practice supports digestion and helps us truly taste and appreciate our food.

Consider your favorite meal—maybe it's a homemade lasagna or a colorful salad. Mindful eating invites us to be curious about the origins of our food, the journey it took to our plate. It's about acknowledging the farmers, the chefs, and the countless hands that contributed to the culinary masterpiece in front of us. Suddenly, each bite becomes a nod of gratitude to the interconnected web of food production.

Now, let's talk about the emotional side of mindful eating. It's like having a conversation with your food, asking yourself, "Am I eating because I'm hungry or for other reasons?" It's about recognizing the difference between physical hunger and emotional cravings, creating a space for a healthier relationship with food.

In a world where speed often trumps presence, mindful eating is a breath of fresh air—a reminder to slow down, savor, and appreciate the simple joy of a good meal. It's not a strict rulebook; it's an invitation to bring mindfulness to the table, transforming eating from a routine into a celebration of life's flavors. So, fellow epicureans, let's put down our forks between bites, relish the textures, and make every meal a mindful adventure. Bon appétit!

THE ART OF SAVORING EACH BITE

An art form that goes beyond the mere act of eating and transforms every meal into a symphony of sensations. Picture this: a dining experience that's not just about consuming calories but about relishing the poetry of tastes, textures, and the sheer delight that comes with every morsel.

Consider your plate as a canvas, and each dish as a unique masterpiece waiting to be explored. This isn't about counting calories or scrutinizing portion sizes; it's about immersing yourself fully in the culinary masterpiece in front of you. It's a dance between you and your plate, where each bite is a step, and the flavors are the music that guides your senses.

In our fast-paced world, meals are often wolfed down like a sprint, the nuances of taste lost in the race against time. The art of savoring is like hitting the pause button. It's about embracing a pace that allows you to truly experience the textures, aromas, and intricate dance of flavors that unfold with every chew.

Imagine walking through a bustling market, surrounded by the vibrant colors and fragrances of fresh produce. Savoring each bite is akin to selecting the ripest fruit, feeling its weight in your hand, and letting the anticipation build before the first taste. It's not just eating; it's an expedition into a world of culinary treasures.

Let's talk about the magic of mindful chewing. Yes, something as simple as chewing. It's not just a mechanical process; it's the first act in the culinary drama within your mouth. The art of savoring encourages us to chew slowly, allowing the flavors to unfold and the senses to engage in a delightful waltz.

Think about your favorite dish. Maybe it's a homemade lasagna or a perfectly grilled steak. Savoring each bite is about exploring the layers of flavors—every herb, every spice, every nuance carefully orchestrated to create a culinary masterpiece. It's not just about tasting; it's about connecting with the craftsmanship behind the dish.

STRATEGIES TO OVERCOME MINDLESS EATING

Conquering mindless eating can be a game-changer in your journey towards a healthier lifestyle. Let's dive into some effective strategies that go beyond diets and restrictions, focusing on cultivating mindfulness and building a positive relationship with food.

1. **Mindful Eating Practices:**

   - **How It Works:** Engage your senses while eating. Pay attention to the colors, textures, and aromas of your food. Chew slowly, savoring each bite.

   - **Why It Helps:** Mindful eating brings awareness to the act of eating, preventing autopilot munching and allowing you to truly enjoy your meals.

2. **Portion Control:**

   - **How It Works:** Use smaller plates and bowls to control portion sizes. Be mindful of serving sizes and avoid going back for seconds without checking in with your hunger cues.

   - **Why It Helps:** Smaller portions help in regulating calorie intake, promoting a balanced and mindful approach to eating.

3. **Create a Dedicated Eating Environment:**

   - **How It Works:** Designate specific areas for eating, avoiding places associated with work or distractions. Sit down at a table and create a relaxed dining atmosphere.

   - **Why It Helps:** Separating eating from other activities reduces mindless snacking and encourages a focused, enjoyable mealtime.

4. **Listen to Hunger Cues:**

- **How It Works:** Tune in to your body's signals of hunger and fullness. Eat when you're hungry, and stop when you're satisfied.

- **Why It Helps:** Listening to your body prevents overeating and fosters a healthier relationship with food.

5. **Food Journaling:**

- **How It Works:** Keep a food journal to track what, when, and why you eat. Note your emotions and circumstances surrounding eating.

- **Why It Helps:** Journaling increases self-awareness, helping you identify patterns of mindless eating and make informed choices.

6. **Snack Mindfully:**

- **How It Works:** When snacking, portion out your snacks, and avoid eating directly from the container. Choose nutritious snacks and savor each bite.

- **Why It Helps:** Mindful snacking prevents the consumption of excess calories and encourages conscious choices.

7. **Plan Balanced Meals:**

- **How It Works:** Prepare well-balanced meals with a mix of protein, healthy fats, and fiber-rich foods. Include a variety of colors and flavors.

- **Why It Helps:** Balanced meals provide sustained energy, reducing the likelihood of mindless snacking on unhealthy options.

8. **Identify Triggers:**

   - **How It Works:** Recognize emotional triggers that lead to mindless eating, such as stress or boredom.

   - **Why It Helps:** Identifying triggers allows you to address the root cause of mindless eating and develop healthier coping mechanisms.

9. **Practice Intuitive Eating:**

   - **How It Works:** Listen to your body's hunger and fullness cues without external diet rules. Allow yourself to enjoy all foods in moderation.

   - **Why It Helps:** Intuitive eating promotes a balanced and sustainable approach to food, fostering a positive relationship with eating.

10. **Stay Hydrated:**

    - **How It Works:** Drink water throughout the day, especially before meals. Sometimes, feelings of hunger can be confused with dehydration.

    - **Why It Helps:** Staying hydrated supports overall well-being and can prevent unnecessary snacking.

Remember, these strategies are not about strict rules but rather about building a mindful, sustainable approach to eating. Incorporate them gradually, and find what works best for you in creating a positive and mindful relationship with food.

SECTION 4

OVERCOMING CHALLENGES

CHAPTER 8

SOCIAL AND ENVIRONMENTAL INFLUENCES

Let's unravel the complex web of social and environmental influences that shape our eating habits. From family gatherings to the layout of our neighborhoods, these factors play a significant role in what, when, and how we eat. So, grab a metaphorical seat at the table, and let's explore the intricacies of our eating landscape.

I. Social Influences:

How It Works: Our social circles, including family, friends, and colleagues, can greatly impact our food choices. Cultural norms, traditions, and social events often shape the types of foods we consume.

Why It Matters: Social influences can either support or challenge our efforts to maintain a healthy diet. Peer pressure, cultural expectations, and communal eating habits can sway our choices.

Possible Solutions:

- **Open Communication:** Discuss your dietary preferences and goals with your social circle. This fosters understanding and support.

- **Potluck Planning:** When gathering with friends or family, organize potluck-style meals, allowing everyone to contribute healthier options.

2. Environmental Influences:

How It Works: Our surroundings, such as the availability of food options in our neighborhoods, workplace environments, and the accessibility of fresh produce, impact our choices.

Why It Matters: Limited access to healthy food options, the prevalence of fast-food outlets, and food deserts can contribute to less nutritious diets.

Possible Solutions:

- **Community Advocacy:** Support and participate in initiatives that aim to bring healthier food options to underserved communities.

- **Office Wellness Programs:** Encourage workplace wellness programs that provide nutritious snacks and meals, promoting a healthy eating culture.

3. Media and Advertising:

How It Works: The constant barrage of food-related advertisements and media influence our perceptions of what is desirable and normal in terms of food choices.

Why It Matters: Misleading advertising, the glamorization of unhealthy foods, and the portrayal of unrealistic body images can contribute to poor dietary choices.

Possible Solutions:

- **Media Literacy:** Educate yourself and others about media literacy, helping to critically analyze food advertisements and make informed choices.

- **Promote Healthier Marketing:** Support campaigns that advocate for healthier food advertising and more transparent labeling.

4. Emotional Influences:

How It Works: Our emotions, stress levels, and mental well-being can significantly impact our eating habits. Emotional eating, often driven by stress or other emotions, can lead to mindless overconsumption.

Why It Matters: Emotional eating can contribute to unhealthy dietary patterns, leading to weight gain and an unhealthy relationship with food.

Possible Solutions:

- **Mindfulness Practices:** Incorporate mindfulness techniques, such as meditation or deep breathing, to manage stress and emotional triggers.

- **Seek Professional Support:** If emotional eating becomes a challenge, consider seeking support from a mental health professional or a registered dietitian.

Navigating the Terrain for Healthier Choices

Our food choices are not made in a vacuum; they are influenced by a myriad of factors in our social and environmental surroundings. Recognizing and understanding these influences empowers us to make informed decisions about our diets. By fostering open communication, advocating for healthier environments, promoting media literacy, and addressing emotional triggers, we can navigate the eating landscape with intention and create a positive, supportive relationship with food. It's a journey worth taking—one that leads to a healthier, happier you. So, let's embrace the challenge, be mindful of our surroundings, and savor the flavors of a balanced and nourishing lifestyle. Bon appétit to a healthier future!

CREATING A SUPPORTIVE ENVIRONMENT

Creating a supportive environment is like planting seeds for a garden of health, where every choice we make is rooted in positivity and vitality. So, let's roll up our sleeves and cultivate a space that uplifts our journey to a healthier, happier life.

1. **Nutritious Nooks in Your Kitchen:**

How It Works: Arrange your kitchen to encourage healthy choices. Keep fresh fruits, veggies, and whole grains easily accessible. Place unhealthy snacks out of sight or better yet, replace them with nutritious alternatives.

Why It Matters: A well-organized kitchen can reduce the temptation of reaching for less nutritious options, making it easier to stick to your health goals.

Possible Solutions:

- **Meal Prep Stations:** Dedicate a space for meal prep with handy tools, making it convenient to whip up healthy meals.

- **Snack Zones:** Create designated areas for wholesome snacks, making it the first choice when hunger strikes.

2. **Active Corners and Fitness Hubs:**

How It Works: Incorporate physical activity into your daily environment. Arrange your furniture to allow for easy movement, set up a home workout space, or keep exercise equipment visible to encourage regular use.

Why It Matters: A physically active environment promotes consistent exercise habits, contributing to overall well-being.

Possible Solutions:

- **Home Workout Zones:** Designate a specific area for exercise equipment or for practicing yoga and other workouts.

- **Active Commuting:** If possible, opt for active transportation methods like biking or walking.

3. Social Support Networks:

How It Works: Surround yourself with a supportive social circle that shares your health goals. Whether it's friends, family, or fitness buddies, having a positive network can significantly impact your well-being.

Why It Matters: Social support provides encouragement, accountability, and shared experiences on the journey to a healthier lifestyle.

Possible Solutions:

- **Join Health-focused Communities:** Participate in online or local groups that align with your health goals, fostering connections with like-minded individuals.

- **Share Your Goals:** Communicate your health aspirations with friends and family, encouraging their support and possibly inspiring them to join you.

4. Mindful Spaces for Relaxation:

How It Works: Create designated areas for relaxation and mindfulness. Whether it's a cozy reading nook, a meditation corner, or a calming bath space, having places to unwind is crucial.

Why It Matters: Stress management is integral to overall well-being, and creating spaces for relaxation supports mental health.

Possible Solutions:

- **Designate Calm Zones:** Create serene areas in your home where you can engage in activities that promote relaxation, such as reading, meditation, or gentle stretching.

- **Incorporate Nature:** Bring elements of nature into your environment, whether through indoor plants, natural light, or calming nature sounds.

5. Positive Environmental Cues:

How It Works: Surround yourself with visual cues that reinforce your health goals. This could include inspirational quotes, images of your fitness journey, or reminders of the benefits of a healthy lifestyle.

Why It Matters: Positive cues serve as constant reminders of your objectives, reinforcing commitment and motivation.

Possible Solutions:

- **Create Vision Boards:** Craft visual representations of your health goals, incorporating images and words that inspire and motivate.

- **Daily Affirmations:** Place positive affirmations in visible areas to encourage a positive mindset and healthy choices.

Cultivating Your Health Oasis

Building a supportive environment is an ongoing process of mindful choices and intentional design. It's about surrounding yourself with elements that champion your well-being and make healthy living the natural choice. Whether it's arranging your kitchen for nutritional success, creating spaces for physical activity and relaxation, or curating a positive social network, every step you take transforms your environment into a haven for health. So, let's plant the seeds of well-being, nurture our health oasis, and watch as it blossoms into a vibrant landscape of vitality. Here's to creating a supportive haven where your health goals thrive and flourish!

SECTION 5

MAINTAINING A HEALTHY LIFESTYLE

CHAPTER 9

BUILDING SUSTAINABLE HABITS

Building sustainable habits that stand the test of time. Think of it as crafting the foundation for a lifestyle that not only supports your health goals but becomes an integral part of who you are. So, grab your metaphorical hard hat, and let's lay down the bricks of sustainable habits, one mindful choice at a time.

I. Start Small, Build Steady:

How It Works: Begin with manageable changes. Small, consistent actions are the building blocks of sustainable habits. Gradually increase complexity as each step becomes ingrained in your routine.

Why It Matters: Starting small reduces overwhelm and allows for gradual adaptation, making it more likely for the habit to stick.

Possible Solutions:

- **Tiny Tweaks:** Instead of overhauling your entire diet, start by incorporating one extra serving of vegetables each day.

- **Micro Workouts:** Begin with short, daily exercises that can easily fit into your schedule.

2. Anchor to Existing Routines:

How It Works: Integrate new habits into established routines. Associating a new behavior with an existing one creates a seamless transition.

Why It Matters: Anchoring to existing routines minimizes disruptions and leverages established patterns for habit formation.

Possible Solutions:

- **Morning Rituals:** Pair a new habit with your morning routine, such as stretching before your morning shower.

- **Mealtime Integration:** Build habits around meals, like taking a short walk after dinner.

3. Mindful Repetition:

How It Works: Consistent repetition reinforces neural pathways, making the behavior more automatic over time. Mindfully engage in the habit to strengthen the connection.

Why It Matters: Repetition forms the basis of habit formation, and mindfulness enhances the learning process.

Possible Solutions:

- **Reflection Practice:** After each repetition, take a moment to reflect on the positive aspects and progress.

- **Visual Cues:** Use visual reminders or habit trackers to reinforce the repetition.

4. Set Realistic Goals:

How It Works: Define clear, achievable objectives for your habits. Realistic goals increase motivation and create a sense of accomplishment.

Why It Matters: Unrealistic goals can lead to frustration and abandonment of habits. Realistic goals build confidence and momentum.

Possible Solutions:

- **SMART Criteria:** Ensure your goals are Specific, Measurable, Achievable, Relevant, and Time-bound.

- **Progressive Targets:** Gradually increase the intensity or duration of your habit as you achieve smaller milestones.

5. Accountability Structures:

How It Works: Share your goals with a friend, family member, or join a community. Having an accountability structure increases commitment and motivation.

Why It Matters: External accountability provides support during challenging times and celebrates successes together.

Possible Solutions:

- **Accountability Partners:** Share your goals with someone who can check in on your progress.

- **Community Engagement:** Join online or local groups focused on building similar habits for mutual support.

6. Adaptability and Resilience:

How It Works: Recognize that setbacks are a natural part of habit-building. Develop resilience by learning from setbacks and adapting your approach.

Why It Matters: Building sustainable habits requires flexibility and the ability to navigate challenges without giving up.

Possible Solutions:

- **Reflect and Learn:** Analyze setbacks to understand their root causes and adjust your approach accordingly.

- **Celebrate Progress:** Acknowledge and celebrate the small victories along the way.

Raising the Structure of Wellness

Constructing sustainable habits is a dynamic process that involves careful planning, mindful repetition, and resilience in the face of challenges. As you lay down each brick, remember that the structure you're building is a reflection of your commitment to a healthier, happier life. So, let's continue to shape our habits with intention, embracing the journey of construction and celebrating the resilient structures of wellness we create along the way. Here's to building a sustainable future, one habit at a time!

MAKING HEALTH A LIFESTYLE, NOT A SHORT-TERM FIX

We're building a lifestyle that echoes with the rhythms of health and happiness. Consider this your blueprint for a sustainable, fulfilling existence where health isn't just a goal but a way of life. So, let's break ground on a foundation that withstands the tests of time and weathers every season with resilience and vibrancy.

****1. Shift the Mindset:**

How It Works: Embrace a mindset that views health as an ongoing journey, not a destination. Shift from temporary fixes to a commitment to continuous improvement.

Why It Matters: A mindset shift lays the groundwork for sustainable habits, fostering a sense of purpose beyond short-term goals.

Possible Solutions:

- **Goal Reframing:** Instead of focusing on quick results, set goals that contribute to long-term well-being.

- **Mindfulness Practices:** Cultivate awareness of the present moment, fostering a deeper connection to your health journey.

2. Nourish with Whole Foods:

How It Works: Prioritize whole, nutrient-dense foods that fuel your body. Build a relationship with food that nourishes and sustains rather than relying on restrictive diets.

Why It Matters: Whole foods provide a comprehensive array of nutrients, promoting overall health and vitality.

Possible Solutions:

- **Balanced Plate Approach:** Design your meals with a variety of colorful fruits, vegetables, lean proteins, and whole grains.

- **Mindful Eating:** Engage in the sensory experience of eating, savoring each bite and paying attention to hunger and fullness cues.

3. Incorporate Joyful Movement:

How It Works: Integrate physical activity that brings joy and fulfillment. Shift from exercise as a chore to movement as a celebration of what your body can achieve.

Why It Matters: Enjoyable movement sustains long-term engagement, making it more likely to become a consistent part of your lifestyle.

Possible Solutions:

- **Explore Various Activities:** Find forms of exercise that resonate with you, whether it's dancing, hiking, or playing a sport.

- **Socialize Through Movement:** Join classes or groups that combine social interaction with physical activity.

4. Prioritize Sleep and Stress Management:

How It Works: Recognize the importance of quality sleep and stress management in overall health. Build routines that prioritize rest and relaxation.

Why It Matters: Consistent sleep and stress management contribute to physical and mental well-being, forming the foundation of a resilient lifestyle.

Possible Solutions:

- **Establish Sleep Hygiene:** Create a calming bedtime routine and maintain a consistent sleep schedule.

- **Mind-Body Practices:** Incorporate activities such as meditation, yoga, or deep breathing to manage stress.

5. Cultivate Supportive Relationships:

How It Works: Surround yourself with individuals who uplift and support your health journey. Foster connections that prioritize well-being.

Why It Matters: Supportive relationships provide encouragement, accountability, and a shared commitment to a healthy lifestyle.

Possible Solutions:

- **Share Goals with Loved Ones:** Communicate your health goals with friends and family, encouraging a collective approach.

- **Build a Support Network:** Join communities or groups focused on health and well-being to connect with like-minded individuals.

6. **Celebrate Progress, Not Perfection:**

How It Works: Shift the focus from perfection to progress. Celebrate small victories and learn from setbacks, recognizing that the journey is dynamic.

Why It Matters: Celebrating progress fosters a positive mindset and resilience, key elements in maintaining a health-focused lifestyle.

Possible Solutions:

- **Reflect Regularly:** Take time to reflect on your health journey, acknowledging achievements and areas for growth.

- **Reward Yourself:** Celebrate milestones with rewards that align with your values and contribute to your well-being.

Crafting Your Health Symphony

Building a lifestyle centered around health is an ongoing symphony of choices, intentions, and celebrations. As you construct this vibrant masterpiece, remember that each note contributes to the harmonious melody of your well-being. So, let's continue to craft a lifestyle that resonates with health, longevity, and joy—a symphony that echoes through the seasons of life. Here's to elevating health into a timeless lifestyle, a melody that plays on, resonating with vitality and fulfillment!

The End

www.ingramcontent.com/pod-product-compliance
Lightning Source LLC
Chambersburg PA
CBHW040110150726
48005CB00013B/1639